Food For Good Health

FOOD SAFETY

Barbara J. Patten, MS

The Rourke Corporation, Inc.
Vero Beach, Florida 32964

PHOTO CREDITS
All photos © Barbara and John Patten

Library of Congress Cataloging-in-Publication Data

Patten, Barbara J., 1951-
    Food safety / Barbara J. Patten.
    p. cm. — (Food for good health)
    Includes index.
    Summary: Discusses how to keep food safe, covering such topics as careful food preparation, different kinds of food poisoning, and the safe packing of lunches.
    ISBN 0-86593-404-5
    1. Food handling—Safety measures—Juvenile literature. 2. Food poisoning—Juvenile literature. [1. Food handling—Safety measures. 2. Safety.] I. Title. II. Series.
TX537.P38   1996
363.19'26—dc20 —dc20   95-33538
                                                                     CIP
                                                                     AC

Printed in the USA

TABLE OF CONTENTS

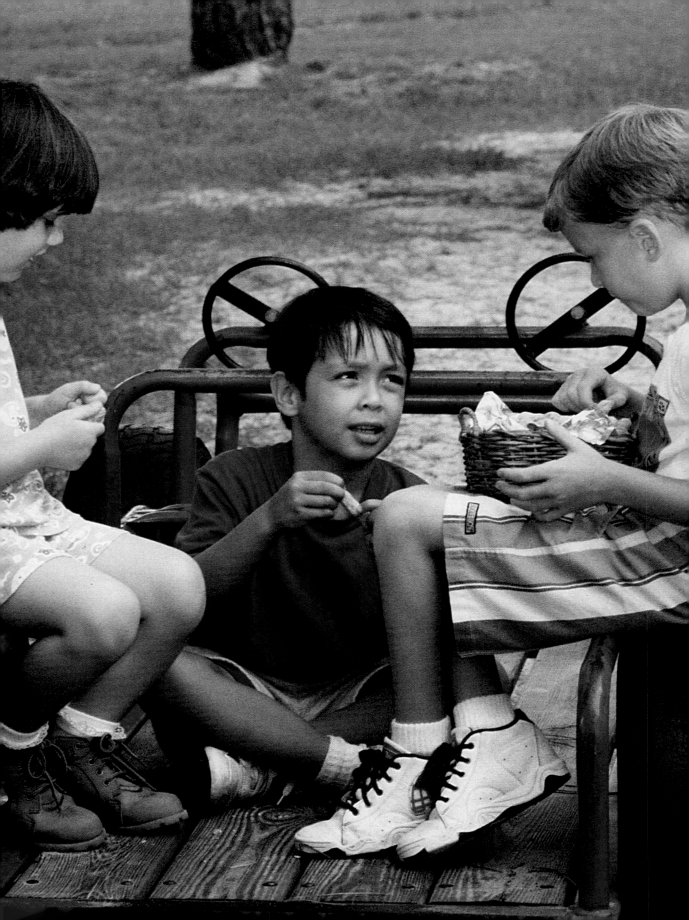

THE FOOD SAFETY PATROL

Food safety is very important. Children who learn how to handle food safely can protect themselves, their friends and their family from sickness.

The three main ideas in food safety are handling and preparing food, avoiding poisons, and eating carefully.

Let's read all about food safety and make you a member of the food safety patrol.

Come join the food safety patrol.

KEEPING FOOD SAFE

Have you ever helped your mom or dad make supper? You can help a lot by finding out about how to keep food safe.

Most of the time, food and water are safe. However, food can become **poisoned** (POY zuhnd), or unsafe to eat, if you store or prepare it in the wrong ways.

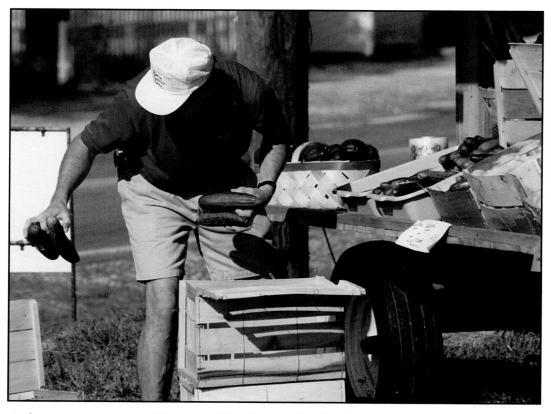

A farmer removes old vegetables from his display.

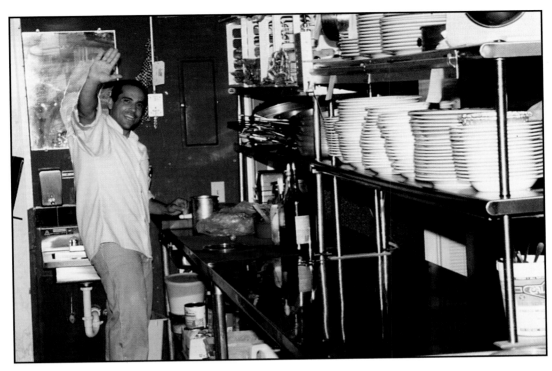

Food safety is important in this restaurant.

Restaurants and grocery stores follow laws that help make sure the foods people buy are safe. People from the government check to see that laws are obeyed.

Still, at home and away, food poisoning is a danger. To be safe, everyone should know the right ways to handle and store food.

FOOD POISONING

Bacteria (bak TEER ee uh), or germs, grow in foods that are old, dirty, under-cooked or not kept cool. These bacteria cause food poisoning.

Food poisoning **symptoms** (SIMP tuhmz), or warning signs, include losing your appetite, vomiting and stomachaches. People with food poisoning stay sick for 12 to 36 hours.

In bad cases of food poisoning, people may have to go to the hospital, and could even die. Very young and very old people get most sick from food poisoning.

Fish can be stored on ice to prevent bacteria growth.

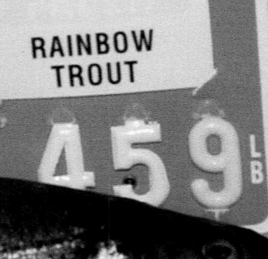

SEAFOOD

FRESH
WHOLE
SNAPPER

$ 389 LB

SEAFOOD

RAINBOW
TROUT

$ 459 LB

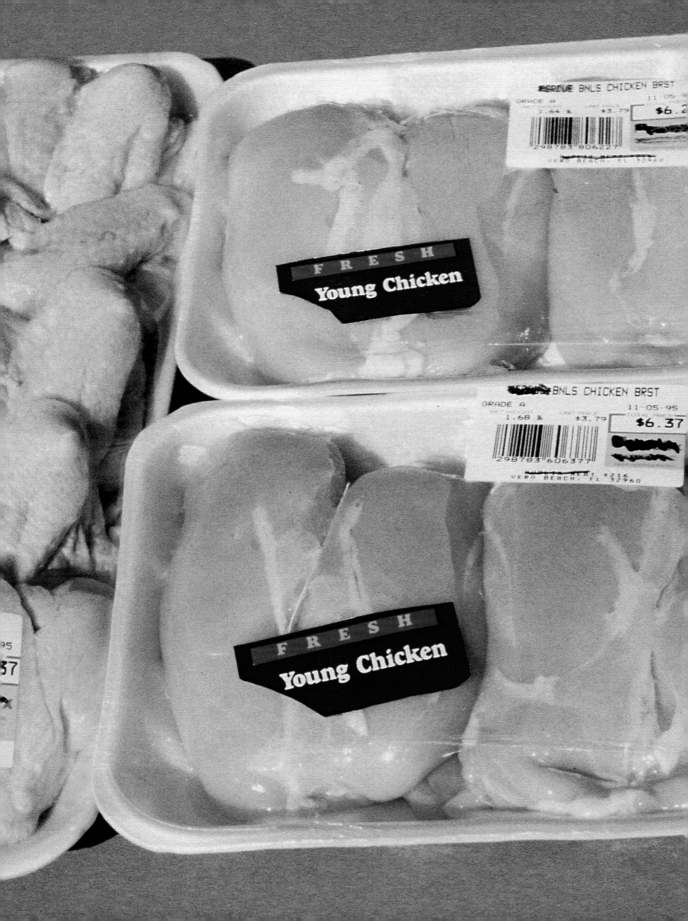

KINDS OF FOOD POISONING

Staph (STAF) is a common food poisoning. Staph bacteria can get in food from dirty hands. Staph grows fast in foods, like meat or milk, that spoil at room temperature.

Salmonella (sal muh NEL uh) bacteria—found in poultry, eggs and meat—causes stomachaches and high fevers. It is a dangerous kind of food poisoning.

You can prevent salmonella by keeping foods cool and cooking them well. Clean up raw food juices from your hands and kitchen tools with soap and hot water.

Salmonella can grow on raw chicken that isn't kept cold.

MORE KINDS OF POISONS

Cooked meat that sits out becomes poisonous. If it's left at room temperature for 12 hours or more, cooked meat becomes unsafe to eat.

Botulism (BOCH uh liz um) is a rare, but dangerous, bacteria that grows in canned foods. You should throw away food you find in bulging or swollen cans.

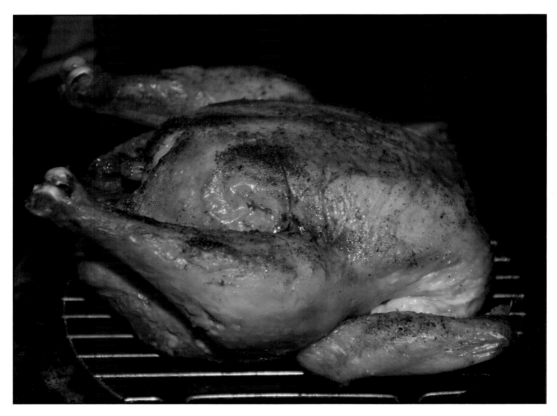

Keep cooked meats in the refrigerator.

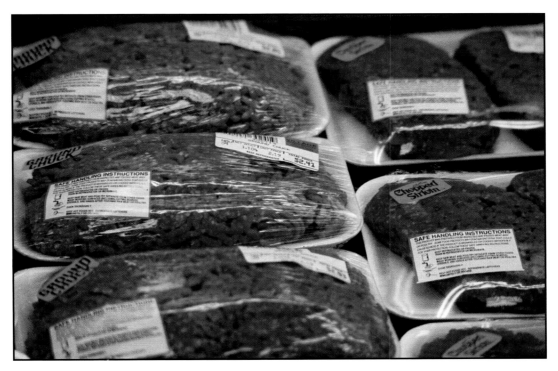
Hamburger should be well-cooked.

Hepatitis A (hep uh TIIT is AY) is a sickness you can get from eating raw oysters and clams that lived in polluted water. Cooked shellfish are much safer to eat.

E. coli (ee KOH lii) are bacteria found in hamburger or ground beef. They die in well-cooked meat. Watch out for burgers that are pink in the middle. They are not cooked through and could have E. coli inside.

BRING A SAFE LUNCH OR SNACK

Are you planning a field trip or picnic? To be safe, take an ice pack or food that won't spoil if you don't keep it cold.

Most meats, milk and salads with mayonnaise spoil quickly if they are not kept cool. Eating foods like these, if they've been left out for a long time, can make you sick.

A peanut butter and jelly sandwich is a good choice for field trips. Washed raw vegetables and fruits won't spoil and are tasty, too. Juice boxes give you a healthy drink in an easy-to-carry way.

Bring a safe lunch or snack on field trips.

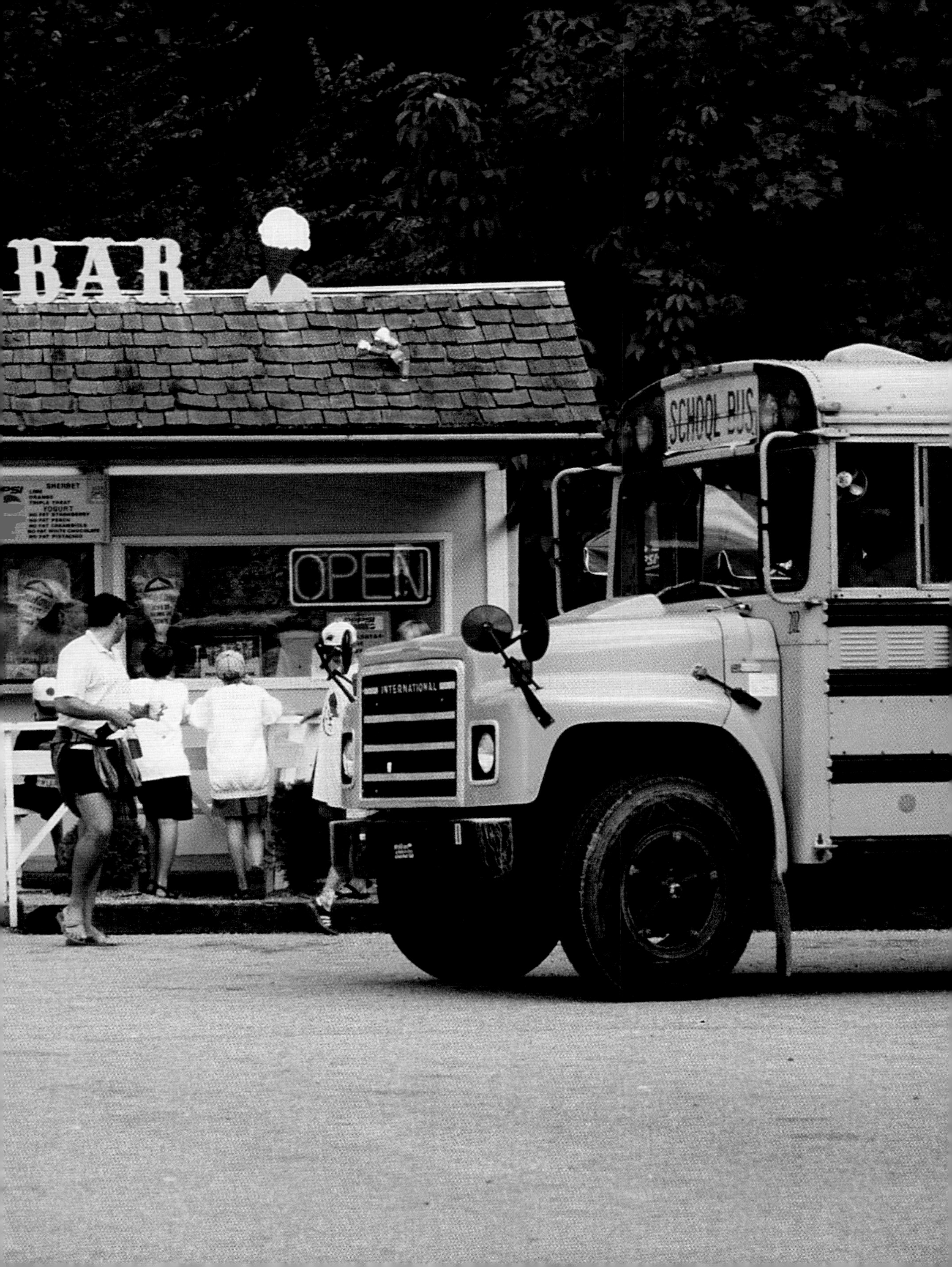
BAR
OPEN
SCHOOL BUS
INTERNATIONAL

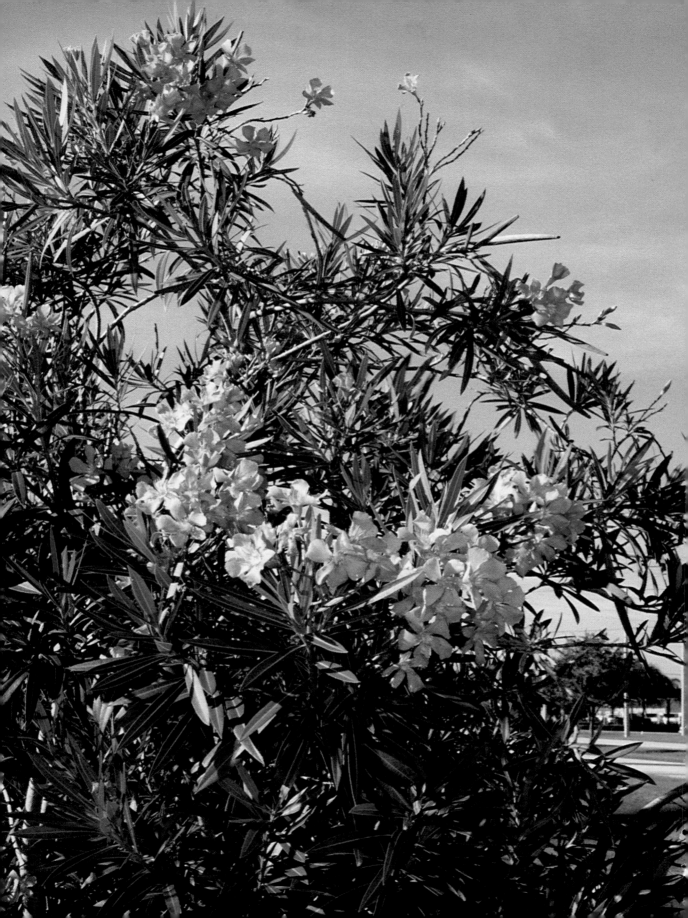

THOSE DANGEROUS PLANTS

Not all plants are good food. Some are dangerous to put in your mouth.

Leaves, berries and flowers from some indoor plants are toxic, or poisonous. You should never taste or play with plants in yards, fields and woods.

Mushrooms that grow outside are not like mushrooms sold in stores. Never eat a wild mushroom because some can be deadly.

The flower, leaf and wood of the oleander are poisonous.

EAT SAFELY—DON'T CHOKE

Sadly, each year adults and children choke to death on food stuck in their throat. You should cut all foods, especially meats, into small pieces and chew them very well.

Choking happens when people try to swallow food pieces that are too big to go down. These pieces get stuck in the throat and cut off the air supply to the lungs.

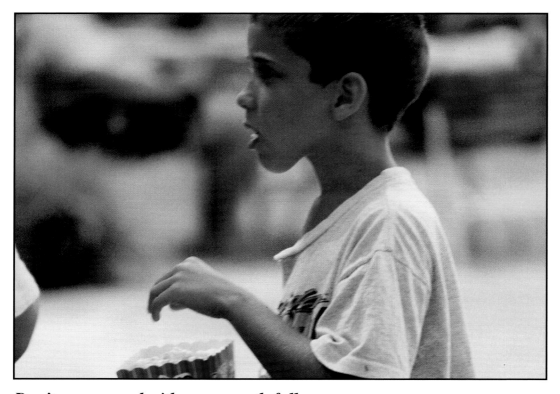

Don't run around with your mouth full.

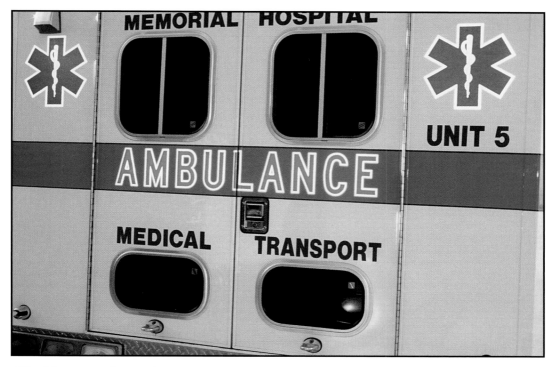

Choking can be serious.

One way to avoid choking is to eat carefully—without running and jumping around with your mouth full.

Also, be extra careful with hot dogs. A hot dog bite is just the right size to plug your throat if you swallow without chewing. If someone is choking, get help right away.

FOOD PATROL SAFETY RULES

Protect yourself and help others. Keep these food safety rules in mind.

Dangerous bacteria can't grow in a clean kitchen or on clean hands. Wash everything that has touched raw meat, fish or poultry with hot soapy water—maybe twice.

Don't let raw or cooked meats, milk, and salads with mayonnaise sit out at room temperature. You should put foods that spoil in the refrigerator right away.

Hamburger, pork, poultry and fish must be well-cooked.

Prevent choking. Eat small pieces and chew them well. Horseplay and eating don't go together.

Dishwashers kill bacteria with very hot water.

20

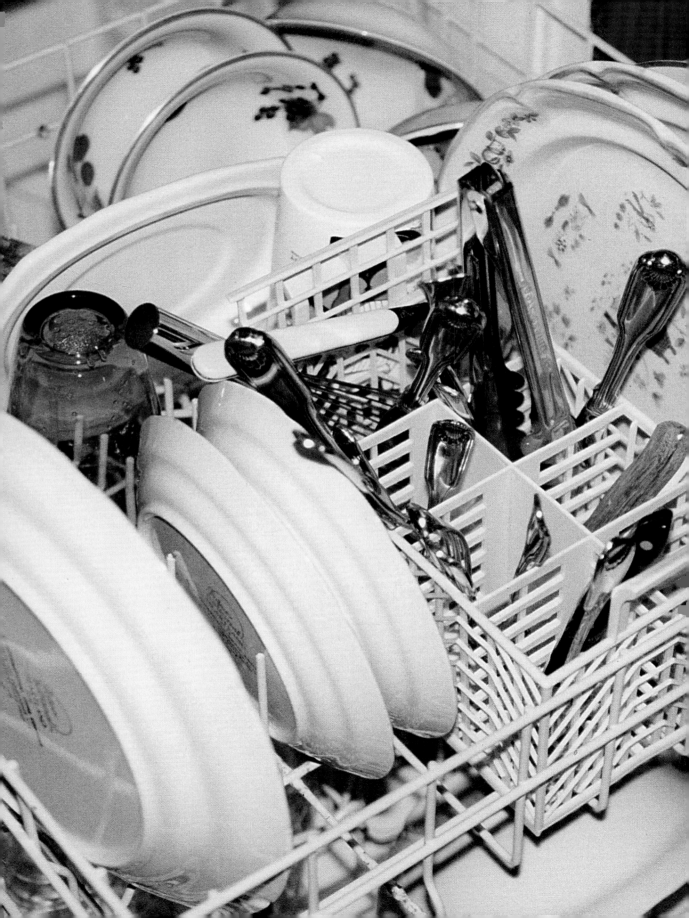

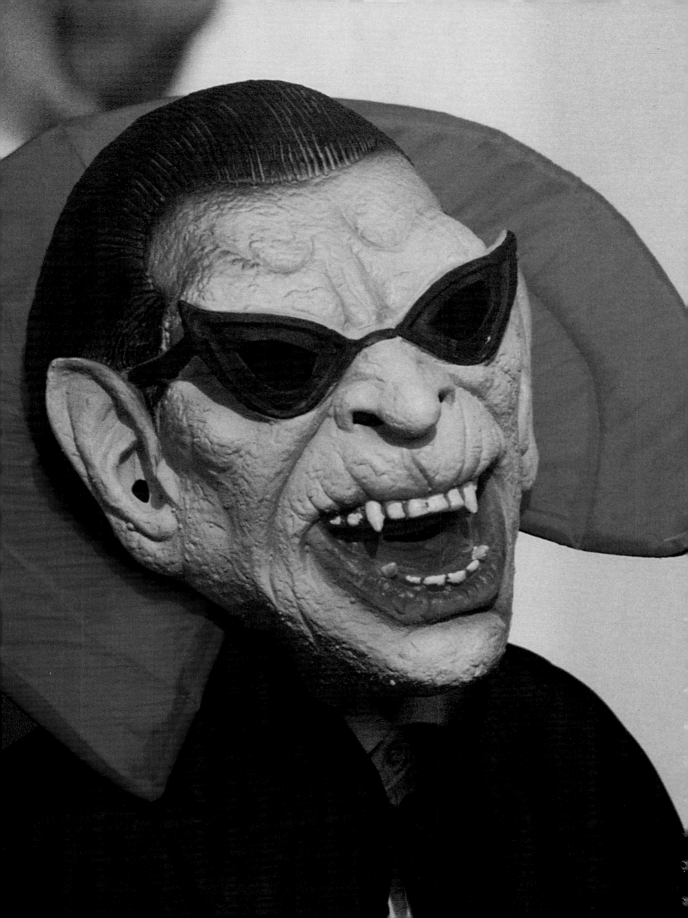

GLOSSARY

bacteria (bak TEER ee uh) — germs

botulism (BOCH uh liz um) — rare but dangerous bacteria

E. coli (ee KOH lii) — bacteria found in hamburger and ground beef

hepatitis A (hep uh TIIT is AY) — a disease caused by eating raw oysters and clams

poisoned (POY zuhnd) — unsafe to eat

salmonella (sal muh NEL uh) — bacteria found in eggs, poultry and meat

staph (STAF) — bacteria that cause food poisoning

symptoms (SIMP tuhmz) — warning signs

Food safety is not a joke.

INDEX

24